THE STRENGTH RECOVERY CLINIC

The Missed Diagnosis

Why your pain keeps coming back

JEAN COCK

Registered Osteopath, M.Ost, BSc (Hons), A-CFMP
Functional Medicine Practitioner

The Missed Diagnosis

Published by The Strength Recovery Clinic

thestrengthrecoveryclinic.com

Registered Osteopath. General Osteopathic Council registration number 10993.

IMPORTANT: PLEASE READ

This guide is general information and education. It is not medical advice, it does not diagnose any condition, and it is not a substitute for individual clinical assessment by a qualified practitioner who has examined you.

Do not start, stop, or change any medication or supplement on the basis of what you read here. If you are taking prescribed medication, are pregnant or breastfeeding, or have a diagnosed medical condition, speak to your GP or pharmacist before making changes.

If you have any of the warning signs listed in the red flag chapter at the back of this guide, seek medical assessment promptly rather than self-managing.

Contents

INTRODUCTION

If you have done everything right and it still hurts

You have done the exercises. You went to physio, possibly more than once. You rested when you were told to rest, and moved when you were told to move. Maybe you had an injection. Maybe you had a scan that came back showing something, or came back showing nothing at all, and neither answer changed how you feel.

And the pain is still there.

The conclusion most people reach at this point is that they are the problem. That they did not try hard enough, or that they are just getting older, or that this is simply how their body is now. I hear this in clinic constantly. People apologise to me for still being in pain, as though they have failed at something.

They almost never have.

In the overwhelming majority of cases where pain has not resolved despite good treatment, the treatment was not wrong. It was aimed at one layer of a problem that has more than one layer. The physio you did was probably appropriate. The manual therapy probably helped, for a while. What was missing was not effort or skill. It was the scope of the investigation.

This guide is about the layers that do not get looked at.

What makes this different

There are excellent books about the psychology of chronic pain and how the nervous system learns to produce it. This is not one of them, and I would encourage you to read them.

What this guide covers is the territory in between. The physical and physiological drivers that sit underneath persistent pain and almost never appear on an assessment form. Internal organs referring pain into the shoulder or the back. Breathing mechanics dictating what the neck has to do twenty thousand times a day.

Blood sugar quietly degrading the quality of every piece of connective tissue your body rebuilds. Inflammation lowering the threshold at which your nervous system decides something is worth telling you about.

None of this is fringe. These are recognised physiological relationships. They get overlooked not because practitioners do not believe in them but because a standard appointment does not have the time to go looking, and because the questions that would reveal them are not on the form.

How to use this guide

Part One explains why persistent pain behaves the way it does. Part Two covers what gets missed. Part Three is a region by region breakdown so you can find your own presentation. Part Four is what to actually do about it, including a chapter on supplements that will probably be more conservative than you expect.

You do not have to read it in order. If you are here because of a specific area, go to Part Three first and work backwards.

One thing before you start. This guide will not diagnose you. Nobody and nothing can do that without examining you and taking your history properly. What it can do is show you what a thorough investigation actually looks at, so that you know what has been missed and what to ask for next.

PART ONE

Why You Are Still In Pain

The problem is rarely effort. It is almost always scope.

CHAPTER ONE

The system was not built for your problem

Modern medicine is extraordinary at acute care. Fractures, infections, strokes, surgical emergencies, trauma. If you are seriously injured or acutely unwell, there is no better system to be inside.

Medicine understands multifactorial disease perfectly well. The problem is not the knowledge. It is the way the system is organised to deliver it.

Care is structured around discrete episodes. One appointment, one presenting complaint, one referral pathway, one specialty. That structure is efficient and it works extremely well when the problem is genuinely contained: a fracture, an infection, an appendix.

Persistent pain is not contained. It sits across musculoskeletal, metabolic, immune, autonomic and psychological territory simultaneously, and the referral system has no pathway that holds all of that in one place. You get sent to the specialty that best matches the loudest symptom, and each specialty investigates its own territory competently and reports back that its territory is clear.

Everyone is 'right'. Nobody has looked at the thing connecting it all, because nobody was asked to and no single appointment was long enough.

The time problem

A new patient musculoskeletal appointment is typically forty-five minutes. A follow-up is around thirty. Inside that window a practitioner has to take a history, examine you, form a working diagnosis, explain it, treat you, and give you something to do at home.

Working through your sleep quality, your digestion, your medication history, your stress load, what your symptoms were doing two years before they became a problem, and whether anything changes after you eat does not fit into that. It is not a question of competence. There is no room.

The questions that are not on the form

The second problem is that even where there is time, the questions that would reveal a non-mechanical driver are not part of a musculoskeletal consultation.

If you present with back pain, you get asked about your back. You are unlikely to be asked whether the pain changes after certain meals, whether your sleep deteriorated before the pain started, whether a new medication coincided with the onset, or whether you have felt gradually less well for considerably longer than you have been in pain.

Those questions take under a minute each. They are simply not on the form.

Symptom suppression is not treatment

There is a related issue worth naming clearly. Reducing a symptom without addressing what is producing or maintaining it may not resolve the problem. It may make the underlying situation harder to detect.

This applies broadly. To painkillers taken for back pain so that you can keep loading a spine that is telling you not to. To maintenance manual therapy that provides genuine relief every few weeks without anything fundamentally changing in between. Pain is information. Silencing it without understanding the reason can interfere with the signal without addressing the problem.

THE DISTINCTION THAT MATTERS

Managed means the pain reduces after a session and returns before the next one. Better means the cause has been identified and addressed, and you have what you need to stay well without permanent dependence on someone else's hands.

If you have been in treatment for a long time and cannot honestly say which of those has been happening, that question is worth sitting with.

DO THIS NOW

Do not walk into your next appointment and describe your symptoms. Everyone does that and it produces the same forty-five minutes you have already had several times. Walk in with a document. Two sides of paper, prepared in advance, containing the things a clinician cannot get from you in the time available.

The onset document

- The date of the first mild version, not the date it became a problem. These are usually months or years apart, and the gap is where the answer often sits
- Everything that changed in the six months before that date. New job, new medication, illness, injury elsewhere, bereavement, house move, dietary change, new exercise, pregnancy, surgery, dental work, infection
- Whether the onset was sudden, gradual, or stepwise with plateaus

The behaviour document

- Twenty-four hour pattern: on waking, at midday, by evening, overnight
- Morning stiffness and precisely how long it takes to ease. Under thirty minutes and over thirty minutes point in different directions
- What position or activity reliably eases it, and how long the relief lasts
- What reliably provokes it, and whether the provocation is immediate or delayed by hours
- Whether it is affected by meals, poor sleep, stress, hot or cold, or the menstrual cycle

The treatment ledger

A table with four columns: what was tried, for how long, what happened, how long the improvement lasted. Include everything, including what you abandoned. A treatment that helped for three days and one that helped for three months are telling you completely different things about the mechanism.

The list nobody asks for

- Every medication, including short courses in the last two years and anything you consider irrelevant, such as antihistamines, acid suppressants, contraception or statins
- Every supplement, with dose
- Every previous investigation and its actual result, in your possession as a document rather than as a memory of what you were told

Hand this over at the start rather than trying to say it out loud. It changes what is possible in the appointment, and any clinician worth seeing will be glad of it.

CHAPTER TWO

Pain is an output, not a location

The instinctive assumption about pain is that it reports damage at the place where you feel it. Sometimes it does. Frequently it does not.

Pain is better understood as an output. Your nervous system continuously integrates information from muscles and joints, from internal organs, from breathing mechanics, from posture and load tolerance, from stress state and autonomic regulation. It weighs all of that and produces a decision about whether to generate pain and where you will feel it.

When one part of that system is persistently irritated, symptoms frequently appear somewhere else entirely. Usually wherever movement or load exposes the weakest link.

Why the sore spot is often not the problem

One of the most reliable rules I work to is that the structures which hurt most are often not the cause of the problem.

That sounds like a platitude until you understand why it is mechanically true.

Tissue becomes painful when the load placed on it exceeds what it is currently conditioned to tolerate. That can happen because the load went up. It can equally happen because the tolerance went down, or because a neighbouring structure stopped taking its share and the load was redistributed.

In the third case, which is common in persistent pain, the tissue that fails is not the tissue that changed. It is simply the least robust structure in the chain at the moment the redistribution happened. It is the weakest link, and the weakest link is where you feel it.

This is why the painful structure is frequently a reliable finding and an unreliable diagnosis. It genuinely is irritated. It is genuinely producing your symptoms. It is not the reason those symptoms exist.

If the shoulder joint itself cannot move properly because the capsule is restricted, the rotator cuff has to work considerably harder to produce the same everyday movements. It becomes sore. It is genuinely the painful structure. It is not the reason.

The same logic applies everywhere. If the shoulder blade is not rotating properly, the space above the rotator cuff narrows every time you lift your arm. If the hips are not taking their share of load during ordinary movement, the lower back takes it instead. These compensations are the everyday mechanical reality of the body, and treating the structure that is complaining without identifying what pushed it into that state is precisely why the pain returns.

> A RULE WORTH REMEMBERING
>
> Most back pain involves sore points on the back. Those sore points frequently have nothing to do with the correct diagnosis. If someone examines you by pressing around until they find something tender and then treats that, they have found a symptom, but not necessarily the cause.

Everything gets treated, nothing changes

This is why the pattern is so recognisable. The disc gets treated. The facet joint gets injected. The muscle gets massaged. Each of those produces a period of relief, because each of those structures genuinely was irritated.

Then it comes back, because the reason they were irritated was never identified.

A forty-five minute appointment, however well intentioned and however skilled the practitioner, cannot assess a system of interacting parts. It can assess a part. If the answer lies in how the parts relate to each other, or in something outside the musculoskeletal system altogether, it will not be found there.

DO THIS NOW

Build a body map with a timeline. This takes twenty minutes and is one of the most diagnostically useful things you can produce.

Step one: the full list

Every area that has hurt in the last five years. Include the ones that resolved. Include the ones you dismissed as minor. Include non-musculoskeletal complaints: headaches, digestive episodes, skin changes, recurrent infections, periods of unexplained fatigue.

Step two: order them

Chronologically, with approximate dates. Mark which resolved fully, which resolved partially, and which are ongoing.

Step three: read the pattern

You are looking for one of four shapes, and each points somewhere different.

- **Single site, recurring.** Points towards an unresolved local mechanical driver, or a loading pattern that has never changed
- **Migrating around the body.** One thing resolves, another appears. Points strongly towards a systemic driver or a global movement strategy problem rather than a series of coincidences
- **Sequential and adjacent.** Foot, then knee, then hip, then back. Points towards a mechanical chain problem propagating upward
- **Widespread and simultaneous, with fatigue.** Points towards an inflammatory, metabolic or central sensitisation picture, and needs medical investigation alongside anything mechanical

Step four: overlay life events

On the same timeline, mark major life events, illnesses, medication changes and periods of high stress. If your musculoskeletal history clusters around those markers rather than around physical incidents, that is the single most important thing you will bring to an appointment.

CHAPTER THREE

Why your pain changes when nothing else has

Some weeks everything hurts more. You have not lifted anything, trained differently, slept badly, or changed a single thing you can identify. The pain is simply worse.

Here is what can be happening, and it is one of the most useful things to understand about your own body.

Often the pain has not increased at all. What has changed is the threshold at which your nervous system decides to tell you about it.

The immune and nervous systems are one system

Your body produces inflammation to protect you. Without that capacity we would not survive long. The immune system is built to identify a perceived threat, deal with it, clear up, and stand down.

What is less widely understood is how closely the immune and nervous systems work together. They function essentially as one integrated survival system, and that system does not only fight infection. It changes your behaviour to help you recover.

The problem arises when that system is triggered constantly rather than occasionally. A persistent low-grade immune response is not strong enough to put you in bed the way a fever would. That is exactly what makes it so easy to miss. What it produces instead, gradually, is a lowering of the nervous system threshold, reduced cellular energy production, altered mood chemistry, and a state of low-level vigilance.

More things register as painful. Sleep gets lighter. Mood dips. Recovery from everything takes longer.

> THIS IS STRATEGY, NOT MALFUNCTION
>
> Every one of those changes increases your chance of survival if your body believes you are under threat. It wants you to withdraw, rest, and recover. A more sensitive nervous system is an advantage when something is trying to harm you. Not dropping into deep sleep makes sense when being unconscious would leave you vulnerable.
>
> The system is doing precisely what it evolved to do. The difficulty is that the threat it is responding to is not what it thinks it is, and it is not switching off.

What this explains

This model helps explain several things that otherwise make little sense.

It explains why your pain flares in a stressful month with no change in physical activity. It explains why two people with apparently identical presentations respond completely differently to the same treatment, one resolving in a single session and the other needing three. It explains why pain can appear to worsen when nothing about the tissue has changed.

Technically, what you are experiencing in these periods is not an increase in pain. It is a sudden awareness of pre-existing pain that your nervous system previously did not consider important enough to report. Now that it is dealing with a sustained load, it needs to be more vigilant, so it tells you. In evolutionary terms that is entirely sensible.

Why this matters for treatment

If the reason your pain became noticeable is a lowered threshold rather than a change in the tissue, then treating the tissue produces exactly what most people describe. Some relief, then a return to where you started.

Manual treatment can reduce a mechanical contribution. It cannot lower a systemic inflammatory load, correct a nutrient deficiency, change what you are eating, or fix a sleep problem that has been running for three years. Where those factors genuinely contribute and remain unaddressed, they can continue to re-prime the system regardless of what is done to the painful area.

That is not an argument against manual therapy. It is a statement about which problems it is the right tool for.

> DO THIS NOW
>
> You are going to run an experiment on yourself for four weeks. The purpose is to find out what your pain actually correlates with, because almost nobody knows and most people are wrong when they guess.
>
> **Record daily, in the evening, ninety seconds**
>
> - **Pain** out of ten: worst point of the day, and average across the day. Record both, they behave differently
> - **Morning stiffness** in minutes, from waking to when it eased
> - **Sleep**: hours, bedtime, number of wakings, and whether it felt restorative on a one to five scale. Restorative quality matters more than duration
> - **Stress** out of ten, plus one word for why
> - **Food**: not everything. Alcohol, anything notably high in sugar or refined carbohydrate, gluten, dairy, and whether you ate late
> - **Movement**: what you did and roughly how much
> - **Bowels**: normal, loose, constipated. More informative than people expect

How to read it after four weeks

Do not look for same-day correlations. Look at a one to two day lag. Inflammatory and sleep-driven pain changes typically show up twenty-four to forty-eight hours after the trigger, which is precisely why people fail to connect them.

- Take your five worst pain days. Look at what the two preceding days looked like
- Take your five best days. Do the same
- Compare the two sets. If sleep, stress or a specific food shows up consistently on one side, you have found something worth acting on
- If pain tracks with physical activity and nothing else, your problem is more purely mechanical than most and should be loaded and progressed accordingly

Bring the log itself, not your summary of it. Four weeks of data changes a consultation more than any description of symptoms can.

PART TWO

What Gets Missed

The layers that are not on anybody's assessment form.

CHAPTER FOUR

When the pain is not coming from where it hurts

This is the chapter I would most want you to read.

Internal organs refer pain into the musculoskeletal system through shared neural pathways. This is called viscerosomatic referral. It is well documented, it is taught, and in my clinical experience it is present far more often than it is identified.

The mechanism is straightforward. Organs and musculoskeletal tissues share spinal cord segments. Irritation or dysfunction in an organ can therefore influence muscle tone, movement, and pain perception in the body wall region that shares those segments. The pain is entirely real and it feels completely mechanical. It behaves slightly differently, which is the clue.

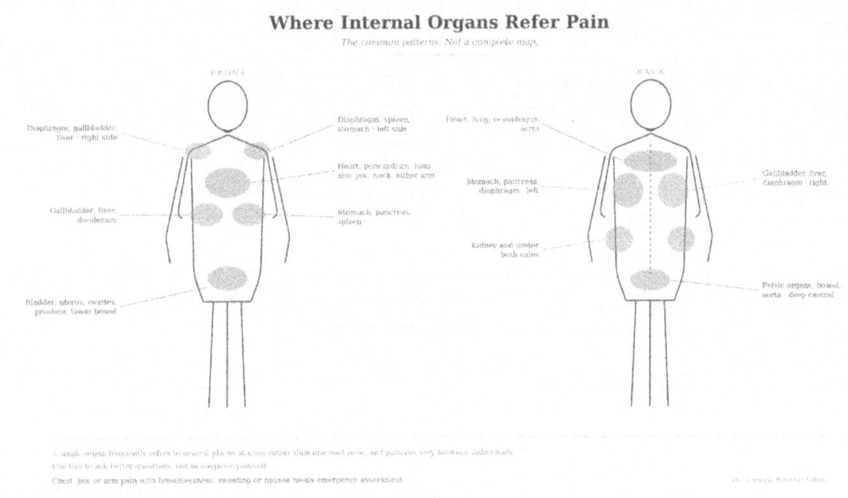

Common viscerosomatic referral zones. Front and back. Not a complete map.

The referral patterns

Structure	Refers to Most common sites, not all	Clue that points to it
Diaphragm	Either shoulder, tip and top. Also the back	Most common visceral driver in my practice. Worse with breathing effort, altered breathing pattern, often bilateral upper trapezius tension
Gallbladder	Right shoulder, right scapula and back	Worse after fatty meals, often delayed by one to three hours. Can be episodic over months
Liver	Right shoulder	Associated with right upper abdominal fullness, alcohol history, medication load
Stomach	Left shoulder, mid back	Relates to meals, reflux, worse lying flat, often mid thoracic stiffness
Spleen	Left shoulder tip	Left upper abdominal discomfort. Sudden onset needs urgent assessment
Pancreas	Left shoulder, mid back	Boring pain through to the back, may ease leaning forward
Lung and pleura	Shoulder, same side. Also the upper back	Changes with deep breathing or coughing rather than with arm movement
Kidney	Flank, low back, groin, shoulder	Less common. Urinary changes, loin tenderness
Heart and pericardium	Chest, either side, jaw, arm	Exertional. Any suspicion needs emergency assessment, not a clinic appointment
Aorta	Deep central abdomen, lower back, flank	Tearing quality, pulsating sensation, feeling faint. Emergency
Pelvic organs	Lower abdomen, low back, sacrum, groin, inner thigh	Uterus, ovaries, prostate, bladder and bowel. Cyclical timing, urinary or bowel change, pain unrelated to movement or load

This list is not exhaustive. Almost every internal structure can refer somewhere in the musculoskeletal system, patterns vary between individuals, and a single organ frequently refers to several places at once rather than one neat zone.

Several structures refer to both sides, including the heart and the peritoneum. It is also worth understanding that the shoulder is only one referral site for these structures. Think about the classic presentation of a heart attack, which can involve the arm, chest, jaw and back simultaneously.

The same principle applies elsewhere. Chronic digestive irritation increases the muscle tone around the mid thoracic spine and raises pain sensitivity across those shared segments. The result is persistent mid-back stiffness that is worse after meals or during stressful periods, with no clear mechanical injury and a normal scan.

The single most useful distinguishing feature across all of these is simple: **visceral referral does not behave mechanically.** Mechanical shoulder pain changes predictably with arm position and load. Visceral referral often does not change much with arm movement at all, but changes with meals, breathing, trunk posture, or time of day. The second feature is that it frequently fails to fully resolve with good mechanical treatment, improves briefly, and returns on a cycle that does not match activity.

> FROM CLINIC
>
> I have seen right shoulder and back pain driven by the gallbladder and diaphragm many times. These two are by far the most common visceral drivers I encounter.
>
> In one case the entire diagnosis turned on a single question: does the shoulder hurt more after a fatty meal? It did, every time, and it had done for months while the shoulder itself was being treated. Nobody had asked.

Breathing, the diaphragm and the shoulder

One of the clearest versions I see is a shoulder that will not respond to rehabilitation.

Someone has done the rotator cuff strengthening. They have done the thoracic mobility work. Load has been adjusted, technique corrected. The pain is still there or keeps returning.

When the whole system is assessed, a contributing driver is sometimes visible within minutes. A paradoxical breathing pattern. A right hemidiaphragm that is barely moving. The entire shoulder girdle compensating with every single breath.

That person is repeating an altered breathing strategy tens of thousands of times every day, including while asleep. No strengthening programme competes with that volume because the pattern repeats continuously.

The diaphragm has direct neurological relationships with the cervical and upper thoracic spine, and autonomic connections influenced by breathing and stress. When breathing mechanics are altered through chronic stress, postural adaptation, or abdominal tension, the shoulder becomes overactive, poorly stabilised under load, and neurologically sensitised. If altered breathing mechanics are maintaining the problem, the shoulder may continue to fail despite good local rehabilitation.

> DO THIS NOW
>
> Two simple self-checks. Neither diagnoses anything, but both produce information worth taking to an appointment.
>
> - **The meal test.** For two weeks, note what you ate and rate your pain three hours later. You are looking for a pattern with fatty meals, large meals, or specific foods. Any consistent link is worth investigating.
> - **The breathing check.** Lie on your back, one hand on your chest and one on your belly. Breathe normally for a minute without trying to change anything. The belly hand should move noticeably more than the chest hand. If the chest hand is doing most of the moving, your breathing mechanics are worth assessing properly.

DO NOT SELF-DIAGNOSE THIS

Visceral referral patterns overlap with symptoms of genuinely serious conditions. Chest, jaw, or left arm pain, particularly with breathlessness, sweating or nausea, needs emergency assessment. New severe abdominal pain, jaundice, blood in stool or urine, or unexplained weight loss needs prompt medical assessment. This chapter is here so you know what to ask about, not so you can conclude it is your gallbladder.

CHAPTER FIVE

The four components of stress nobody assessed

The word stress has been used so loosely for so long that it has lost most of its meaning.

Ask someone whether they are stressed and the overwhelming majority will say they are fine. They are not being dishonest. They are answering a question about how they feel emotionally, which is roughly a quarter of what stress actually is, and the part their body is least likely to be struggling with.

The four components

Understood properly, stress has four components operating at the same time.

Component	What it means in practice
Psychological and emotional	Work, relationships, finances, caring responsibilities, unresolved history
Inflammatory	Diet, gut function, infections, environmental exposures, unresolved injury
Circadian disruption	Poor or irregular sleep, shift work, light exposure at the wrong times
Blood sugar dysregulation	Insulin resistance, glucose swings, long gaps then large meals

In many people, more than one of these is present simultaneously. The combined physiological effect is not something that can be treated away with manual therapy or exercise, no matter how well either is delivered.

What this looks like in a shoulder

The clinical consequences are both direct and indirect.

Directly, inflammatory conditions such as polymyalgia rheumatica can produce pain and stiffness across the shoulder and hip girdles, and symptoms may be unlikely to resolve sustainably while the systemic inflammatory process remains active. No amount of treatment to the shoulder changes this.

Indirectly, consider adhesive capsulitis, commonly called frozen shoulder. Most people treat it as a purely musculoskeletal condition. It is not. It is associated with hormonal imbalance, metabolic conditions including diabetes and hypothyroidism, cardiovascular disease, post-surgical complications, and some neurodegenerative conditions. Treating it as a local shoulder problem without considering those contributors can leave important maintaining factors unaddressed.

Why you did not notice

Human beings are poorly calibrated for gradual change. We rationalise, normalise, sit in denial, self-justify, and have genuinely unreliable memories for how we used to feel.

That combination almost guarantees we miss exactly the changes we most need to notice. It is why so many people accept as normal that they are more tired, have less energy, feel weaker, think less clearly, and are more irritable than they were five years ago.

I want to be clear about this. That decline is common. That does not make it normal, and it is not an inevitable function of age.

> DO THIS NOW
>
> Score yourself honestly out of ten on each of the four components, where ten is maximum load. Most people who believe they are not stressed score low on the first and considerably higher on the other three.
>
> Then pick the highest scoring one and identify a single change you could sustain for six weeks. One change, held consistently, outperforms five changes abandoned in a fortnight.

CHAPTER SIX

Your tissue is only as good as what builds it

Muscle, bone, fascia, tendon and cartilage are all biological material. Your body is constantly breaking them down, recycling them, and rebuilding them, provided it has the resources and the conditions to do so.

What you eat, how you sleep, your inflammatory load and your metabolic health all determine the quality of what gets rebuilt. This is not a wellness idea. It is the basic reality of tissue turnover, and it has direct consequences for pain.

Repair under inflammation

Ongoing inflammation can alter tissue remodelling and repair, particularly when it is persistent and combined with other factors that impair recovery. The tissue is more fibrotic, less flexible, and more prone to further injury. The body does not get a period of relative calm in which to reorganise it properly.

This is one reason people wake up stiff. The more of this that has accumulated, the stiffer the morning, and in some cases the stiffness persists all day. Marked morning stiffness is also a feature of active inflammatory conditions, which is one reason it should be taken seriously rather than accepted as ageing.

Glycation, in plain terms

Glycation is the process by which a sugar molecule bonds to a protein molecule. It happens continuously, and the rate at which it happens depends heavily on blood sugar regulation.

The analogy is crude but useful. Stick your fingers in honey and they become tacky and cling to one another; glycation does something very similar to proteins, including structural proteins such as collagen, and accumulated glycation can affect tissue properties over time. You can see the same process in ageing skin, where it alters the structure of collagen.

The consequence is that the tissue is compromised before it has done anything. It sustains damage more readily, becomes inflamed more easily, and does not have the mechanical properties it should.

> WHY THIS MATTERS FOR YOUR SCAN
>
> Two people can have identical degenerative findings on imaging and completely different outcomes, because the rate at which their tissue is degrading and their capacity to repair it are not the same.
>
> Being told that a disc shows wear and that this is normal for your age is only half the picture. The question nobody asks is why it is wearing faster than it should be.

The blood test problem

The most common experience people describe is having bloods taken, being told everything is normal, and still feeling unwell.

Usually the tests were not wrong. The issue is that standard reference ranges are wide, the panel requested is limited, and the ranges themselves are derived from population data that includes plenty of people who are not well. A result inside the range is not the same as a result that is optimal for you.

Blood sugar is the clearest example. HbA1c reflects average glucose over roughly the preceding three months. It tells you very little about insulin, and insulin resistance can be present for years while HbA1c sits comfortably inside the normal range. By the time glucose crosses a diagnostic threshold, metabolic dysfunction may already have been developing for some time.

QUESTIONS WORTH ASKING YOUR GP

First, always: ask for the actual numbers, not to be told they are normal. You are entitled to them. Then ask where each sits within the range rather than simply whether it is inside it.

Thyroid: TSH alone is not a thyroid panel

Most people are screened with TSH only. TSH is a pituitary hormone. It tells you what the pituitary is asking for, not what is actually available to your tissues or whether it is being converted properly.

- **TSH**, as the starting point
- **Free T4**, the storage hormone
- **Free T3**, the active hormone. Rarely run and frequently the informative one
- **Reverse T3**, which competes with T3 and rises under physiological stress and illness
- **TPO and thyroglobulin antibodies**, which can be raised for years before any hormone level moves, and which change the whole clinical picture

Iron: four markers, not one

Ferritin alone is not an iron panel and is genuinely misleading in isolation, because ferritin is an acute phase reactant and rises with inflammation. Someone inflamed and iron deficient can show a perfectly reassuring ferritin.

- **Serum iron**
- **Ferritin**, stores, interpreted alongside an inflammatory marker
- **TIBC or transferrin**, total iron binding capacity
- **Transferrin saturation**, the ratio that distinguishes deficiency from overload and is the marker most often missing

Ask for CRP at the same time. Without it you cannot interpret ferritin.

Blood sugar: three markers, not one

- **HbA1c**, average glucose over roughly three months
- **Fasting glucose**
- **Fasting insulin**, almost never run in routine practice, and the one that shows how hard your body is working to keep glucose normal. Insulin rises years before glucose does

Also worth having

- **Vitamin D**, and **B12 with folate** together, since they interact
- **Full blood count** with red cell size, which points towards which deficiency is likely
- **CRP**, and **ESR** where an inflammatory condition is being considered
- **Calcium and magnesium**, particularly before anyone suggests you supplement either

Keep every result. A single snapshot tells you far less than the same marker tracked over three years.

CHAPTER SEVEN

The scan that answered the wrong question

Imaging is a tool. It is not a diagnosis, and treating it as one produces poor outcomes with considerable reliability.

A substantial body of research shows that structural findings on imaging, including disc bulges, degenerative change and rotator cuff tears, are frequently present in people with no pain at all. The reverse is equally true. People with significant and disabling pain often have entirely unremarkable imaging.

The scan shows what is there structurally. It cannot tell you whether what it shows is what is causing your symptoms.

When imaging is actually indicated

For musculoskeletal presentations there are broadly two situations where imaging is appropriate as a primary investigation. Where there is clinical suspicion of a red flag condition, and where an appropriate course of conservative treatment has genuinely failed.

Outside those situations, early imaging can produce more problems than it solves. It anchors everyone to a finding that may be incidental, and it can make you afraid of your own spine.

> A CASE THAT ILLUSTRATES THE COST
>
> A patient came to me with nerve symptoms down the arm and an old disc bulge at C5/6 on a previous MRI. Repeat scans had been ordered on the strength of that finding.
>
> The actual clinical picture included swelling of the arm and hand, warmth, dilated vessels and intermittently cold fingertips. Swelling and temperature change are not features of nerve root compression. They point to a neurovascular mechanism, which was what was going on.

> The scan finding became the entire focus of management and the real diagnosis was missed for years while the condition worsened. That is not a rare failure. It is what happens when imaging substitutes for clinical reasoning.

What this means for you

If you have a scan report, it is worth understanding what it does and does not establish. Degeneration on a report does not mean your pain is explained. It means degeneration is present, which by middle age is extremely common and frequently asymptomatic.

When a scan result and the clinical picture disagree, the clinical picture should generally win.

> DO THIS NOW
>
> - Request a copy of your imaging report if you do not have one
> - Ask specifically: does this finding explain my symptoms, and how do you know?
> - Ask whether the finding would be expected in someone my age without pain
> - If the answer is vague, that is useful information in itself

PART THREE

Region By Region

Find your presentation, and what usually sits underneath it.

CHAPTER EIGHT

Lower back pain

Lower back pain is one of the most common presentations there is and one of the most poorly managed. The reason is usually not a lack of treatment but a lack of precision about what is being treated.

There is rarely a single cause. Most mechanical back pain involves two or more of the patterns below operating together.

One point before the list. Serious pathology is a rare cause of lower back pain. Around ninety-nine percent of cases are musculoskeletal rather than sinister. The remaining one percent involves infection, malignancy, fracture, cauda equina syndrome, etc. Those require urgent assessment and should not be self-managed, which is what the red flag chapter at the back of this guide is for.

Why mechanical back pain is rarely just mechanical

The traditional model of back pain as a purely structural problem is increasingly insufficient on its own. In clinical practice the picture has changed. Chronic low-grade inflammation, gut dysfunction, visceral referral, metabolic dysfunction and systemic disease are now commonly present alongside what presents as straightforward mechanical back pain. They are not always the primary driver, but they are present often enough that ignoring them produces exactly the pattern most people with persistent back pain already know: treatment that helps temporarily and never fully resolves it.

The viscerosomatic relationship described in Chapter Four is one of the most consistently overlooked mechanisms here. Internal organs and spinal structures share neural pathways. Irritation or dysfunction in a visceral structure can increase muscle tone, alter joint mechanics, and produce or maintain pain in the corresponding spinal region. A tight lower back that appears entirely mechanical but does not fully respond to mechanical treatment is worth investigating from that angle. In practice it is increasingly common: restricted lower backs that respond only partially to spinal treatment but resolve more completely when the gut, the kidney or the pelvic viscera are assessed and addressed alongside the musculoskeletal work.

This does not mean every back pain has a visceral cause. It means that assessing back pain as an isolated mechanical problem, without considering what else may be maintaining it, produces incomplete results in a significant and growing proportion of people. The six patterns below remain the essential framework. They should be applied in the context of the whole system rather than in isolation from it.

Disc herniation and discogenic pain

Either the disc bulges and presses on a nerve root, producing leg pain with possible pins and needles, numbness or weakness, or the disc is irritated without significant bulging and produces back pain alone. Typical features include morning stiffness, difficulty putting on socks and shoes, and intolerance of prolonged sitting. Many acute disc-related problems improve substantially within several weeks, although recovery varies with the presentation, severity and the wider factors affecting recovery.

What tends to help: if you have leg pain, gently explore the direction that eases the leg symptoms. For a disc this is usually extension, bending backwards. If that helps, two sets of ten repetitions every four hours for a week is a reasonable trial. If it does not help, or if there are no leg symptoms, avoid prolonged sitting, keep walking, and use ice for no more than fifteen minutes at a time. Keep everything under four out of ten on your pain scale.

Facet joint syndrome

The small paired joints at the back of each segment. Typically one-sided pain, difficulty with transitional movements such as turning in bed or getting up from a chair, often a preference for sitting over standing, and sometimes relief from leaning slightly forward.

What tends to help: a posterior pelvic tilt, gently flattening the lower back against a surface, tends to open the facet joints and reduce the pain. More importantly, learning to rotate through the hips rather than twisting through the lower back alone makes an immediate difference in most people with this presentation.

Sprains and strains

Usually the result of overstretching a fatigued, weak or tight muscle, either in one movement or through repetition. Pain on stretch or activation, sometimes with swelling, stiffness or spasm. Rarely occurs in isolation: there is often a movement, loading or preparation factor that contributed to the conditions in which it occurred.

What tends to help: gentle regular movement within a comfortable range, soft tissue work, and ice in the acute phase. Graded return to loading once the acute phase has settled, with attention to the movement quality that contributed to the injury in the first place.

Spondylosis

Degenerative change. Stiffness first thing that eases within about half an hour, discomfort after sustained positions, and reduced range of movement. Remember that these findings on imaging do not predict symptoms.

What tends to help: consistent movement is the most important factor, because sustained loading in one position is what drives the stiffness. Graded progressive loading, strength work appropriate to your current capacity, and addressing the postural and movement factors that contribute tend to produce the best outcomes over time.

Sacroiliac joint dysfunction

One-sided low back or buttock pain, sometimes referring to the knee, with difficulty bending, sitting, walking on uneven ground or climbing stairs.

A common misconception, in clinical practice and in patient education alike, is that sacroiliac dysfunction is mainly about how much or how little the joint moves. Research consistently shows that movement there is minimal in healthy people, typically a few millimetres of translation and a few degrees of rotation. Focusing on the quantity of movement misses what the joint is actually for. It sits at the intersection of the spine, the pelvis and the lower limbs, and its role is to absorb, distribute and transmit load between them.

This is better understood through tensegrity, the idea that structural integrity depends on balanced tension and compression across interconnected tissues rather than on rigid compression alone. The joint behaves as a node in a continuous network of bone, ligament, fascia and muscle. Anything that disrupts the balance across that network, whether weakness, asymmetry, injury or altered movement, changes how force is transferred through the joint and can produce pain regardless of how much it is moving.

What tends to help: the distinction that matters is how the joint is being loaded, not how far it travels. Where the joint has stiffened and is not sharing load, muscle energy techniques restore normal mechanics. A simple version: lie on your back, bring the affected leg to ninety degrees at the hip and knee, place your hand on the knee, and push the knee into your hand for eight seconds with no movement occurring. Relax and repeat four to six times. Where the supporting system is not controlling load well, the priority is stability instead: strengthening the core and the glutes, and changing the movement patterns that repeatedly stress the joint.

Spinal instability and hypermobility

Ligaments held long over time lose some of their passive support capacity. The nervous system compensates by increasing muscle tone. The result is chronically tight muscles protecting an unstable segment. Stretching those muscles gives temporary relief and does not address why they tightened, which is why the cycle continues for years.

The mechanism is worth understanding properly. Ligaments connect bone to bone and provide passive support. Held in a lengthened position over time they creep, meaning they take longer to return to their resting length. Someone who sits for long periods will typically have posterior spinal ligaments that are longer than their standing posture requires, which leaves the segment relatively unstable and the muscles working to hold it.

What tends to help: stability work rather than stretching. Strengthening the deep stabilisers of the spine and pelvis under load, improving the movement patterns that repeatedly strain the affected ligaments, and building the active support capacity of the whole system around the unstable segments.

GENERAL PRINCIPLES FOR MECHANICAL BACK PAIN

- Find a position that eases things and build movement out from there
- Keep everything under four out of ten on your pain scale
- Identify and remove the specific daily triggers. This is often the single most effective step
- Do not become fear-avoidant. Move as much and as normally as you can within that limit
- Use the hips rather than twisting through the lower back during transitions

CAUDA EQUINA: GO TO A&E, DO NOT WAIT

These are the specific questions that should be asked of anyone with back pain and are frequently not. Any one of them warrants emergency assessment on the same day. Do not wait to see whether it settles.

Bladder. Difficulty starting urination. A sense that the bladder is full but you cannot empty it. Loss of the sensation that tells you that you need to go. Not feeling the urine passing. Leaking without knowing.

Bowel. Loss of control. Not being able to feel a bowel movement passing. Loss of the urge to go. New constipation that feels different from dietary constipation.

Saddle sensation. Numbness, tingling or altered sensation anywhere that would contact a saddle: buttocks, inner thighs, genitals, around the back passage. A useful test is whether wiping after using the toilet feels normal. If it feels different or you cannot feel it, that is significant.

Sexual function. New loss of genital sensation, or new erectile dysfunction alongside back pain.

Legs. Weakness, numbness or pain affecting both legs, particularly if it is worsening.

Symptoms may develop over hours or over a few days. Not all of them need to be present. One or two together are enough to require emergency assessment, and treatment within twenty-four hours is strongly associated with better recovery.

CHAPTER NINE

Neck pain

Neck pain is a musculoskeletal presentation but it is rarely a purely mechanical problem. Viscerosomatic connections between the diaphragm, the lungs and the cervical spine, dural tension, fascial continuity from the thorax into the neck, breathing mechanics, stress hormones and metabolic factors all contribute in ways a structurally focused assessment will miss entirely.

Cervical facet joint syndrome

Each cervical segment has two facet joints at the back which guide and limit movement. They become painful through a combination of inflammation, degenerative change and altered loading. Poor postural habits, weak deep cervical stabilisers, ligament laxity and sustained positions that compress the facets all contribute over time.

Typically one-sided. Worse looking over the shoulder or extending the neck. Morning stiffness or stiffness after rest that eases with movement. Often a dull ache into the shoulder or upper back. Neurological symptoms are not typical of pure facet pain, but can occur where facet enlargement narrows the space through which a nerve root exits.

Referral patterns are predictable. Upper cervical facets refer towards the head and occiput and contribute to cervicogenic headache. Mid-cervical refer into the shoulder and upper trapezius. Lower cervical refer towards the scapula.

What tends to help: addressing the loading pattern matters more than treating the joint. Forward head posture, weak deep neck flexors, thoracic stiffness forcing the neck to compensate, and sustained compression from sitting. Gentle movement in a non-provocative range, heat, and postural correction first. Strengthening the deep stabilisers reduces the mechanical demand over time. Where inflammatory load is high, addressing diet, sleep and metabolic health reduces the background sensitisation that makes facet pain disproportionate to the stimulus.

Cervical radiculopathy

A nerve root compressed or irritated as it exits the spine, most commonly C6 or C7. C6 typically produces symptoms along the lateral forearm into the thumb and index finger. C7 into the middle finger and sometimes the triceps and posterior forearm.

The directional behaviour is clinically important and is frequently recorded imprecisely. Discogenic radiculopathy is typically worsened by neck flexion and positions that increase disc pressure. Facet-mediated foraminal compression is typically worsened by extension and rotation towards the affected side. Both can be relieved by placing the hand on top of the head, which reduces tension on the nerve root, but the provocative directions differ and help identify the primary driver.

Metabolic factors matter here too. Diabetes, insulin resistance and glycation can affect nerve repair capacity and increase susceptibility to compressive neuropathy. Someone with underlying metabolic dysfunction may become symptomatic from a degree of compression that would be subclinical in a metabolically healthy person, and will recover more slowly without that picture being addressed.

What tends to help: positions and movements that reduce nerve root tension, activity modification to avoid compressing the affected foramen, and progressive loading as symptoms settle. Most cervical radiculopathy responds well to conservative management given time. Persistent or progressive weakness warrants further investigation.

Discogenic pain without radiculopathy

A cervical disc can be irritated, inflamed or degenerating without compressing a nerve. Pain is localised to the neck and possibly the upper back or shoulder, without the arm symptoms of radiculopathy. Stiffness with certain movements, discomfort after prolonged sitting or sustained head positions, and headaches arising from cervical muscle tension. Morning stiffness and pain after inactivity are common.

What tends to help: avoiding sustained provocative positions is the most immediately useful step. Gentle movement within a comfortable range, progressive loading as tolerance improves, and addressing the postural patterns loading the disc repeatedly. Most settle within six to twelve weeks with appropriate management.

Ligamentous hypermobility and instability

Cervical ligaments provide passive support. When overstretched through injury, chronic posture or constitutional hypermobility, the joints they support become relatively unstable. The nervous system compensates by increasing muscle tone, producing the tight, guarded neck that never fully relaxes regardless of how much treatment it receives.

This is the same mechanism as the spinal instability described in the back pain chapter. Stretching a cervically unstable neck provides temporary neurological relief while potentially reinforcing the underlying instability. Presentations range from persistent tightness and fatigue through to more significant instability producing dizziness, visual disturbance, and a sense of the head feeling heavy or unsupported. The latter warrants careful assessment before any treatment.

What tends to help: stability work rather than stretching or passive mobilisation. Strengthening the deep cervical flexors and the muscles supporting the cervicothoracic junction, improving postural control, and identifying what is perpetuating the ligament strain. Slower than treating acute neck pain, and considerably more durable.

Muscular trigger points

Hyperirritable spots within muscle that produce local pain, restricted movement and referred pain in patterns that can convincingly mimic nerve root compression.

- **Scalenes:** refer into the chest, upper back and lateral arm into the thumb and index finger, closely mimicking C6 radiculopathy or thoracic outlet syndrome. Dysfunction here also affects breathing and rib mechanics
- **Upper trapezius:** lateral neck, behind the ear, into the temple. A major contributor to cervicogenic headache. Strongly associated with sustained shoulder elevation from desk work and stress
- **Levator scapulae:** deep aching along the medial border of the scapula and posterior neck, worse with rotation or side bending
- **Suboccipitals:** refer into the head and behind the eye

These commonly occur alongside postural overload, sustained positions, repetitive use and chronic stress. Treating them without addressing the cause produces improvement that recurs.

Cervical spondylosis

Degenerative change including disc degeneration, facet osteoarthritis, osteophyte formation and ligamentous thickening. Extremely common after forty and frequently present with no symptoms at all.

Where symptomatic: chronic stiffness, reduced range, discomfort after sustained positions, referred pain into the upper back or shoulders. Where osteophytes narrow the neural foramina, radiculopathy may develop. Where the spinal canal narrows significantly, the cord itself can be affected, which is covered in the red flag box below and is the presentation that must not be missed.

Imaging findings of spondylosis do not predict symptoms. Treating the scan rather than the patient produces poor outcomes.

What tends to help: consistent movement and progressive loading appropriate to current capacity. Avoiding sustained compression in provocative positions. Addressing inflammatory and metabolic load matters particularly here, since glycation and poor blood sugar regulation may contribute to cartilage and disc degeneration.

Thoracic outlet syndrome

Compression of the nerves or blood vessels passing through one or more of three spaces: the scalene triangle between the anterior and middle scalenes, the costoclavicular space between the clavicle and first rib, and the subcoracoid space beneath the pectoralis minor tendon. More than one site is often involved simultaneously.

The neurogenic form is most common and produces pain, tingling, numbness and weakness in the arm and hand that can closely resemble cervical radiculopathy. Additional features that point away from a purely nerve root problem include coldness or colour change in the fingers, swelling of the arm or hand, visible vein distension, and muscle fatigue or cramping with use.

Those vascular features matter enormously. Swelling and temperature change are not features of nerve root compression. If they are present, the mechanism is not simply a disc.

What tends to help: addressing the underlying motor control problem, improving thoracic and cervical posture, releasing the scalenes and pectoralis minor, restoring first rib mobility, and correcting the movement patterns perpetuating the overload.

ALSO SEEK URGENT ASSESSMENT

Severe unrelenting neck pain at rest or at night. Neck pain with unexplained weight loss, fever or night sweats. Neck pain following significant trauma. Sudden severe neck or occipital pain with dizziness, visual disturbance, slurred speech, difficulty swallowing or facial numbness, which requires emergency assessment. Neck pain with a history of cancer, or with long-term steroid use, or in anyone with inflammatory arthritis affecting the upper cervical spine. The screen for sudden severe neck or occipital pain is the 5 Ds, 3 Ns and 1 A: dizziness, diplopia (double vision), dysarthria (slurred speech), dysphagia (difficulty swallowing), drop attacks, nausea, numbness, nystagmus (flickering eye movements) and ataxia (loss of coordination).

CERVICAL MYELOPATHY: THE ONE THAT GETS MISSED FOR YEARS

Compression of the spinal cord itself, as opposed to a nerve root. It is frequently missed because the early symptoms are vague and get attributed to age. The onset is typically insidious and progresses in a stepwise fashion. Prognosis is significantly worse once symptoms have been present beyond about eighteen months, which is why recognising it early matters so much.

Hand function is often the earliest sign. Not weakness, but clumsiness. Difficulty with buttons, zips, keys, handwriting. Dropping things. Fumbling coins. Patients rarely describe this as weakness, they describe it as being clumsy, and it therefore gets dismissed.

Gait and balance change. Feeling unsteady. Walking with a wider base than you used to. Reduced walking speed and shorter stride. Reaching for walls or furniture. Family members often notice this before the patient does. Difficulty walking heel to toe in a straight line.

Bilateral symptoms. Numbness or altered sensation in both hands, rather than one arm in a single nerve distribution. Symptoms that do not follow a clean dermatomal pattern.

Later features. Urinary urgency, hesitancy or incontinence. Stiffness or spasticity in the legs.

Any combination of hand clumsiness, unsteady gait and bilateral hand symptoms in someone with neck pain needs neurological examination and imaging. Do not accept this being attributed to getting older.

CHAPTER TEN

Shoulder pain

The standard narrative around shoulder pain is remarkably narrow. Almost everything gets attributed to the rotator cuff, arthritis, degeneration or age.

The shoulder is the most mobile joint in the body and that mobility has a cost. Unlike the hip, which sits deep in a socket, the shoulder is essentially a golf ball balanced on a tee. The socket is shallow and covers only a fraction of the head of the humerus at any moment. Stability therefore depends almost entirely on soft tissue rather than on bone.

The four rotator cuff muscles exist primarily to hold the head of the humerus centred in that socket while the larger muscles generate force. When they are not doing that job well, the head of the humerus migrates upward and forward during movement and compresses the structures above and in front of it. That is one important mechanical mechanism behind rotator cuff and impingement problems.

Five reasons a shoulder does not get better

One: the whole complex has not been assessed

The most common failure and the most straightforward to fix. Bursitis misdiagnosed as rotator cuff dysfunction. Degenerative change mistaken for capsular restriction. AC joint pathology presenting as biceps tendinopathy. Rotator cuff symptoms driven by a scapula that is not rotating properly. Scapular dysfunction driven by a thoracic spine that will not move. Shoulder pain originating entirely from the cervical spine.

The rotator cuff gets blamed for almost everything, partly because it is the most familiar structure and partly because a proper whole-complex assessment takes longer than most appointments allow. It is frequently symptomatic because something else created the conditions for it to be overloaded.

In my clinical experience many shoulder presentations have a significant cervical spine component. Shoulder pain that has not responded to shoulder treatment is worth assessing from the neck first.

Two: it is not coming from the shoulder at all

Viscerosomatic referral, covered in Chapter Four. The diaphragm and gallbladder are among the most common visceral drivers I see. If your shoulder pain does not change much with arm position but does change with meals, breathing or time of day, that pattern needs investigating rather than treating.

Three: stress, in all four of its forms

Covered in Chapter Five. Two specific applications matter here. Inflammatory conditions such as polymyalgia rheumatica produce shoulder pain that will not resolve until systemic inflammatory load is reduced, regardless of manual treatment.

And adhesive capsulitis, frozen shoulder, is not a purely musculoskeletal diagnosis despite being treated as one almost universally. It has recognised associations with diabetes, thyroid dysfunction, hormonal imbalance, cardiovascular disease, post-surgical states and some neurodegenerative conditions. Treating it locally without investigating those is a significant part of why it takes so long and why it recurs.

Four: nobody took a proper history

The case history often provides the most important diagnostic information. The examination exists to confirm or refute what the history has already suggested. Relying on hands and orthopaedic tests without a thorough history is a guess, and in a shoulder, where referral patterns are this varied, it is a guess with a poor success rate.

Temporary relief is not resolution. If you have felt better for a few days or weeks after each session and then returned to baseline, the mechanism may not have been identified.

Five: imaging was used as the diagnosis

Covered in Chapter Seven. Rotator cuff tears are extremely common in people with no shoulder pain whatsoever. Finding one on a scan does not establish that it is producing your symptoms.

> **SEEK URGENT ASSESSMENT**
>
> Shoulder pain with chest tightness, breathlessness, sweating or nausea needs emergency assessment. Shoulder pain with jaundice, severe abdominal pain or fever needs prompt medical assessment. A shoulder that cannot be lifted at all after trauma needs assessment for a significant tear or fracture.

CHAPTER ELEVEN

Hip pain

Most people with persistent hip pain have already done the sensible things. Physiotherapy, sometimes several courses. Steroid injections. Rest when told to rest. In some cases they have been told surgery is next.

The pain either returns or never fully goes.

The hip is often treated in isolation even when important contributing factors sit elsewhere. The lower back loading into it. The opposite leg not taking its share. The pelvis under load during ordinary walking rather than during a clinical test.

Your hip is rarely the problem

After working with a significant number of people whose hip pain has failed to resolve, the pattern is consistent. The hip is usually the victim rather than the cause. It is the structure that ends up overloaded and symptomatic because something upstream or downstream is not doing its job. Most persistent hip pain falls into one of three patterns, and knowing which one applies changes the whole approach.

Front hip pain that is worse with sitting and stairs

Pain at the front of the hip when getting up from sitting, climbing stairs, or putting on shoes. It is commonly labelled impingement or wear and tear. The socket and the head of the femur are not moving smoothly together, but that is rarely the primary cause. More often the lower back has stiffened and the hip is compensating by working harder than it should, the core is not stabilising the pelvis adequately, and sustained sitting has shortened the hip flexors and altered the joint mechanics. Treating the hip while the back and the core are left alone means the load never changes, so the pain returns.

Outer hip ache that is worse lying on it or walking uphill

A persistent ache on the side of the hip, often worse lying on that side at night, walking on uneven ground, or standing on one leg. It is typically labelled trochanteric bursitis or gluteal tendinopathy. The underlying issue is usually gluteal weakness. The muscles that should be controlling the leg during walking and single leg stance are not doing it, so the tendon and the bursa are repeatedly compressed and irritated. An injection reduces the inflammation and leaves the mechanical cause entirely intact, which is why it comes back.

Deep buttock ache that travels down the leg

A deep, diffuse ache in the buttock that sometimes travels into the thigh or the leg. It is worse with prolonged sitting, bending forward, or walking for long periods, and it is often labelled sciatica or written off as referred from the lumbar spine. In most cases both are involved: the deep hip rotators irritating neural structures and the lumbar spine referring into the same region. Treating only the back or only the hip misses the interaction between the two, which is why the symptoms persist.

Why standard treatment keeps failing

Conventional rehabilitation follows a logical sequence. Identify the painful structure, load it progressively, and send the person home with exercises. For an acute injury that works well. For persistent hip pain it almost always falls short, because the hip does not function in isolation. Its mechanics are influenced by the lower back, the pelvis, the opposite leg, the core, and the way the whole body loads during ordinary movement. When one part of that system is not working properly the rest compensates, and over months and years those compensations, rather than the original injury, are what drive the symptoms.

A forty-five minute assessment focused on the hip alone cannot identify a problem at that level. The examination has to look at the whole movement chain, and the treatment has to address the drivers rather than the site of the pain.

Why injections often disappoint

A steroid injection reduces inflammation. It does not address whatever produced the inflammation. If the loading pattern that overloaded the tissue is unchanged, the tissue will be overloaded again once the injection wears off. The relief was real. The cause was untouched.

The systemic layer

Everything in Part Two applies here with particular force. A hip carrying a mechanical load it was not built to carry alone, in a body with elevated inflammatory load and poor sleep, has both a mechanical problem and an impaired capacity to recover from it. Treating only the first half explains a great many disappointing outcomes.

There is a group of factors that a standard assessment never addresses and that determine whether tissue heals. In people whose hip pain has persisted for a long time, these are almost always present to some degree.

- **Chronic stress and raised cortisol** increase systemic inflammation and reduce tissue healing capacity. Someone under sustained stress does not recover at the same rate as someone who is not, regardless of how well they do their exercises.
- **Sleep disruption** impairs repair directly. Most healing happens during sleep. Poor quality sleep, even when the hours look adequate, means the body is not getting the recovery time it needs between loading sessions.
- **Subclinical inflammation** driven by diet, gut health or metabolic dysfunction keeps pain sensitivity elevated and makes tissue less tolerant of load. People in this state flare easily, recover slowly, and never quite reach a stable baseline.
- **Hormonal change,** particularly in perimenopause and beyond, affects tendon integrity, joint laxity and pain thresholds in ways that are rarely factored into a musculoskeletal assessment.

These are not alternative ideas. They are established physiological mechanisms that affect outcomes and that a thorough assessment should be accounting for.

WORTH ASSESSING IF YOUR HIP KEEPS FAILING

- How the lower back and pelvis are moving during ordinary walking, not just on a couch
- Whether the opposite leg is contributing normally
- Single leg control and balance on both sides
- Foot mechanics, since what happens at the ground travels upward
- Sleep, inflammatory load and metabolic health, which determine repair capacity

THIS IS WORTH INVESTIGATING PROPERLY IF

- The hip pain has been present for months or years without fully resolving
- Physiotherapy has helped temporarily but the pain always returns
- Injections have given short-term relief and the problem has come back
- Scans are normal, or show only mild changes that do not explain the level of pain
- Symptoms fluctuate noticeably with stress or sleep quality
- Several structures have been treated without lasting improvement

SEEK URGENT ASSESSMENT

Inability to weight bear after a fall, particularly in older adults or anyone with osteoporosis. Hip pain with fever. Night pain that is severe and unrelenting. Unexplained weight loss alongside hip pain.

PART FOUR

What To Actually Do

Remove the drivers, then rebuild the capacity.

CHAPTER TWELVE

Reduce the triggers first

Before any technique, exercise or supplement, the single most valuable thing you can do is identify what is driving the problem day to day and reduce it.

When the triggers are removed and the body is being used more efficiently, the need for most of the other interventions falls away substantially. The body often regulates and adapts well when the conditions maintaining the problem are removed.

The most common example there is

The desk worker with a neck that tightens no matter how much it is stretched. The real drivers are almost always screen height, mouse position, chair setup, and hours of sustained forward head posture. These are low-level mechanical triggers operating for eight hours a day.

Address them and the neck has no mechanical reason to stay tight. The stretching was managing a symptom that the environment was recreating every single day.

Triggers are not always mechanical

This is worth stating plainly because it is where most people stop looking.

I once saw a builder with shoulder and leg pain and regular headaches that had been present for over thirty years. He had seen an osteopath more than a hundred times across that period without lasting improvement, and had put it down to age and the physical demands of his work.

Taking a full history made it clear that his diet was heavily reliant on gluten. Sandwiches, pasta, bread at most meals. Two weeks after removing it completely his pain was gone, his energy had returned, and he described feeling like a different person.

That is one person and it is not a universal rule. Gluten does not cause shoulder pain. The point is that his driver was systemic rather than mechanical, and no amount of manual treatment was ever going to resolve a systemic driver. Accurate identification of the cause changes everything.

DO THIS NOW

Spend two weeks auditing rather than treating. Two audits, run at the same time.

The mechanical audit

- Every sustained position the painful area is held in for more than twenty minutes, and the daily total in hours
- Every repeated movement it performs, and roughly how many times per day
- Your workstation, measured rather than estimated. Screen top relative to eye level, elbow angle at the keyboard, whether your forearms are supported, feet flat or dangling
- How you sleep. Position, pillow height, mattress age, and whether you wake in a different position from the one you started in
- Your commute, your bag, which shoulder you carry it on, your shoes

The food and symptom audit

This is the one most people skip and it is frequently the one that finds the answer. You are not counting calories and you are not eliminating anything yet. You are looking for a delayed relationship.

- Record everything you eat and drink, with rough timings
- Record pain out of ten, morning stiffness in minutes, energy, bloating and bowel pattern
- Note alcohol separately, and note anything eaten within three hours of bed

Read it with a lag. Food-related symptoms can sometimes appear with a substantial delay, which is one reason people may fail to connect them. Take your worst three days and look at the two days before each of them. Do the same for your best three days.

The most common repeat offenders in my experience are gluten-containing foods, dairy, alcohol, and high refined carbohydrate meals, but the point is not to assume. The point is to find your pattern.

If a pattern appears, that is the point at which a structured elimination and reintroduction is worth doing properly, ideally with support rather than by guesswork, because done badly it produces unnecessary restriction and no clear answer.

Then act

Change the single largest item from either audit. One thing. Hold it for six weeks before judging it. Changing five things at once means you will never know which one mattered.

CHAPTER THIRTEEN

What to do instead of stretching

Muscle tightness can be a protective response to instability, threat, overload or altered movement rather than a problem in its own right. Passive stretching addresses the sensation while leaving the reason intact, which is why the tightness returns.

What follows tends to work better. None of it suits every situation. If something does not help after a fair trial, it is the wrong tool for what is actually going on.

Trigger pointing

Find the tender, grainy or nodular spot with a thumb, ball or roller. Apply steady pressure at a tolerable level, around six or seven out of ten, breathing slowly. Hold thirty to ninety seconds until the sensitivity eases, then retest the movement. Three to five spots per muscle group. Avoid pressing over nerves, bony points, bruising or swelling, and stop if pain sharpens or shoots.

Foam rolling

Useful as a warm-up or to replace static stretching before activity. Be clear about what it does: the effect is largely neurological rather than structural, creating a short window in which movement feels easier. That window is useful if you follow it immediately with purposeful movement. On its own the effect is short-lived. Roll slowly for sixty to ninety seconds, pausing twenty to thirty seconds on tender areas, avoiding the lower back and bony areas.

Muscle energy techniques

Move to a comfortable barrier. Contract the target muscle gently against light resistance at around twenty to thirty percent effort for five to ten seconds. Relax fully, take up the new slack, repeat three to five times. Precise positioning matters far more than effort.

Reciprocal inhibition

Contracting one muscle can reduce neural drive to its functional antagonist. If the hip flexors feel tight, eight to twelve slow controlled glute bridges will often produce an immediate sense of ease in hip extension without stretching the hip flexors at all. Simple, quick, and badly underused.

Progressive strengthening

This is what makes the change last. In most chronic tightness, the tight area is being asked to do more than it is currently conditioned for. Two to three sessions a week of targeted strength work in the relevant area, progressed gradually, changes load tolerance and reduces the protective drive over time.

> THE SEQUENCE THAT WORKS
>
> Reduce the triggers. Use a technique above to create a window of easier movement. Follow it immediately with purposeful movement. Build progressive strength so the improvement holds. In that order.

CHAPTER FOURTEEN

Movement retraining and body awareness

Proprioception can become less reliable with injury, inactivity, ageing and repeated movement patterns. It is your brain's sense of where your body is in space and how much force is travelling through it.

You notice it as tripping more than you used to, missing kerbs, general clumsiness, feeling unsteady on uneven ground. What you do not notice is that the same loss is quietly changing how you move in ways that feel entirely normal while setting up the next injury.

The clearest example

Knee pain with a foot arch that collapses slightly on every step. Thousands of repetitions a day, and because the feedback from the foot is poor, the nervous system may not adequately correct it. That small repeated collapse changes how force travels up into the knee every time.

Treat the knee all you like. If the foot keeps collapsing the same way, the knee keeps complaining.

The same principle applies to a shoulder irritated by a shoulder blade that is not moving properly, a lower back flaring because the hips are not doing their share, or an ankle that keeps rolling because balance was never fully restored after the first sprain years ago.

The four stages of retraining

Stage	What it involves
Identify the pattern	Not where it hurts, but how you actually move in the activities that matter. Requires watching movement, not just examining tissue

Stage	What it involves
Restore the feedback	Balance work, single leg control, slow controlled movement through avoided ranges. Attention and control rather than repetition
Build on it	Add load and complexity gradually once the pattern is reliable. This is where resilience actually gets built
Apply it	The real test is whether the new pattern appears in walking, stairs and picking things up, not whether you can do the exercise

A STARTING POINT

Two minutes a day, barefoot, somewhere you can steady yourself if needed.

- Stand on one leg for thirty seconds each side, eyes open. Progress to eyes closed only when this is genuinely easy
- While standing on one leg, notice what the foot is doing. Can you feel the arch? Can you keep it from collapsing without gripping with your toes?
- Slow controlled step-downs from a low step, four to six each side, watching that the knee tracks over the middle of the foot

Slow and attentive beats fast and repetitive here. The point is the quality of the signal, not the number of repetitions.

CHAPTER FIFTEEN

The repair environment

You can do everything right mechanically and still not recover if the environment your body is repairing in is working against you.

Sleep

Sleep is a major period for tissue repair, recovery and regulation of pain sensitivity. Poor sleep lowers your pain threshold, which means the same problem hurts more, and reduces your capacity to repair the tissue that is causing it. Both directions at once.

If you improve one thing on this entire list, make it sleep. Consistent timing matters more than total duration for most people. Light exposure in the morning and reduced light in the evening supports the circadian signal that drives the whole system.

Food and inflammatory load

The aim is not a restrictive diet. It is reducing what is provoking an ongoing immune response and providing what is needed to rebuild tissue.

In practical terms that means adequate protein, since you cannot rebuild connective tissue without the raw material. It means not being afraid of fat. It means paying attention to your total carbohydrate load and to how your own body responds to it rather than assuming something is fine because it is generally regarded as healthy. Repeated glucose spikes contribute to the glycation described in Chapter Six.

Movement

Most people are considerably less active than their bodies are built for, and a good proportion of the activity they do involves the same faulty patterns discussed in Chapter Fourteen.

This produces a difficult position. In pain, told to move more, and afraid that moving will make it worse. Sometimes, because the pattern has not changed, it does. That is a reason to retrain the pattern before loading it, not a reason to stay still.

> THE FOUR THAT MAKE THE MOST DIFFERENCE
>
> - Consistent sleep and wake times, held for at least six weeks before judging
> - Protein at every meal, and enough of it
> - Daylight in the first hour after waking, outdoors, even briefly
> - Daily movement below your pain threshold, every day, rather than intense sessions twice a week

CHAPTER SIXTEEN

Supplements: test first, then decide

This chapter is going to be more conservative than you might expect, and there is a good reason for that.

Supplements are not a shortcut around the rest of this guide. They are useful in one specific circumstance: correcting an identified insufficiency that is genuinely limiting your recovery. Taking things speculatively because they are associated with pain or inflammation is expensive, occasionally harmful, and makes it impossible to work out what is actually helping.

> THE SINGLE MOST IMPORTANT PRINCIPLE
>
> Test first. Then decide.
>
> Without testing you are guessing, and with several nutrients guessing carries real risk. Iron is the clearest example and it is covered below.

Iron: never supplement it blind

This is the one I want you to take most seriously, because getting it wrong causes harm rather than simply wasting money.

Iron deficiency and iron overload both produce fatigue, and they require completely opposite responses. Excess iron accumulates in tissue and is genuinely damaging. Haemochromatosis, the commonest genetic cause of iron overload, is more common in northern European populations than most people assume and is frequently undiagnosed for years.

Ferritin alone will not tell you which situation you are in, because ferritin is an acute phase reactant. It rises with inflammation. Someone who is both inflamed and iron deficient can produce a ferritin result that looks entirely reassuring while their actual iron stores are low.

Ask for the full panel: serum iron, ferritin, TIBC or transferrin, and transferrin saturation, which is the marker that most reliably separates deficiency from overload and is the one most often left off. Ask for CRP at the same time, because without an inflammatory marker you cannot interpret the ferritin.

If you supplement iron, it should be because a test showed you needed it, and it should be rechecked.

Calcium: the one people take for the wrong reason

This deserves its own section because the pattern is so common and so counterproductive.

People are told they have osteopenia or osteoporosis, they buy calcium, and they stop there. The belief is that calcium will rebuild the bone. It will not, on its own, and taking it in isolation is not a neutral act.

Bone is living tissue that responds to load. One important intervention for bone density is progressive resistance training and impact appropriate to your situation. Calcium is a raw material. Supplying raw material to a construction site with nobody working on it does not build anything.

Calcium also does not operate alone. Its handling depends on vitamin D status, vitamin K2, and magnesium. Supplementing calcium in isolation, particularly at high doses, without knowing your existing status is not something to do casually, and there is ongoing debate in the literature about cardiovascular risk with high-dose isolated calcium supplementation that has not been settled.

Check your calcium level, your vitamin D, and ideally your parathyroid hormone before anyone puts you on calcium indefinitely. And load your skeleton, because that is the part that actually changes the outcome.

Whole food sources over isolated nutrients

A principle worth understanding: nutrients in food arrive in combination, and those combinations often matter.

Cod liver oil is a useful illustration. It contains vitamins A and D together with omega 3 fatty acids. Vitamins A, D, E and K are fat soluble and interact with one another in the body, so obtaining them together in a food matrix behaves differently from taking an isolated high-dose vitamin D tablet. The same logic applies to desiccated liver, which supplies iron, B12, vitamin A and folate together rather than in isolation.

That is an argument for preferring food-based sources where they suit you. It is not an argument that they are risk-free. Both cod liver oil and liver contain substantial vitamin A, which is fat soluble, accumulates, and matters particularly in pregnancy. Both need the same caution about knowing your iron status.

Where there is reasonable discussion, and the caveats

Nutrient	What is discussed, and what to be careful about
Magnesium glycinate form	Widely discussed in relation to sleep quality and muscle tension. Glycinate is generally better tolerated than oxide, which is poorly absorbed and tends to act as a laxative. The glycine component is itself discussed in relation to sleep. Caution with reduced kidney function, where magnesium accumulates. Timing matters if you take certain antibiotics or thyroid medication, since it interferes with absorption.
Vitamin B12	Absorption requires adequate stomach acid and intrinsic factor. Low stomach acid becomes more common with age and is associated with long-term acid-suppressing medication, which is a recognised reason for insufficiency despite an adequate diet. This is why B12 can be low in someone whose intake looks fine on paper. Test B12 alongside folate, since they interact, and be aware that serum B12 can appear adequate while function is not.

Nutrient	What is discussed, and what to be careful about
Vitamin D	Insufficiency is common in the UK, particularly through winter. Cheap to test, so test rather than assume. Fat soluble and accumulates, so high doses should not run indefinitely without rechecking. Interacts with calcium handling and with vitamin K2.
Omega 3	Discussed extensively in relation to inflammatory load. Affects bleeding time, which matters if you take anticoagulants or have surgery approaching.
Creatine	One of the most studied supplements there is, primarily for muscle. Relevant here because maintaining muscle mass supports load tolerance and bone. Requires adequate hydration.

BEFORE YOU BUY ANYTHING

Speak to your GP or pharmacist first if you take any prescribed medication, are pregnant or breastfeeding, have kidney or liver disease, or have a diagnosed medical condition. Interactions between supplements and medication are real and are frequently overlooked.

Nothing in this chapter is a recommendation to take anything. It is a description of what is discussed in this area and what to be careful about. Your situation requires assessment, not a list.

A SENSIBLE ORDER OF OPERATIONS

- Fix sleep, protein intake and daily movement first. These are the foundations to address before adding more interventions, and they cost nothing
- Test before supplementing. Particularly iron, and particularly calcium
- Prefer food sources where they suit you, since nutrients arrive in combination
- Change one thing at a time, or you will never know what worked
- Give it eight to twelve weeks before judging
- Retest rather than assuming
- If you are on prescribed medication, check interactions with a pharmacist before you start anything

CHAPTER SEVENTEEN

How to get properly assessed

The most important skill in any clinician you see is the ability to diagnose safely and accurately. Without it, everything else is a guessing game that may work in the short term and can go badly wrong.

What a thorough assessment covers

Most of the information needed comes from the history rather than the examination. The examination exists to confirm or rule out what the history has already suggested.

A thorough history covers what happened and when, how function is affected, whether it is improving or worsening, the quality and pattern of symptoms, what makes it better and worse, whether it has happened before, what has already been tried, and what your daily and occupational demands actually are. Alongside that: previous injuries, illnesses, surgery, investigations, current and past medication, family history, alcohol and smoking, diet, sleep and exercise.

Then the systemic questions that usually get skipped: cardiovascular and respiratory, ENT, endocrine and hormonal, digestive, bowel and bladder, urogenital, psychosocial and stress load, and general wellbeing including sleep, energy and headaches.

Two people can present with what looks like identical calf pain. One is mechanical, one is vascular. What separates them at first contact is whether the right questions were asked.

Questions you are entitled to ask

1. What is my diagnosis, and how confident are you in it?
2. What is the prognosis and the expected timeframe?
3. What are the alternatives to what you are proposing?

4. What are the risks, benefits and side effects?
5. Can I have a second opinion?
6. Can I have a copy of my clinical notes?

You can always bring someone with you. You can always withdraw consent. If consent was never properly obtained before examination or treatment, you are entitled to ask why.

Signs it may be time to find someone else

- Regular maintenance sessions with no clear rationale or end point
- No diagnosis offered or explained
- No reassessment despite months or years of treatment
- No curiosity about why the problem exists or what maintains it
- No treatment plan with a goal and a timeline
- Your triggers, movement, sleep, diet and lifestyle have never been discussed
- No exercises or anything practical to do between sessions
- The same treatment repeated despite no meaningful progress
- Your questions are unwelcome

> THE DISTINCTION WORTH MAKING
>
> There is a difference between a good clinician and a practitioner you like. A comfortable, friendly relationship feels good and it is not the same as good clinical care.
>
> Good care makes you more autonomous, not more dependent. You should leave understanding what was happening, why, and what to do about it.

Red flags: when to stop and seek assessment

Nothing else in this guide applies if any of the following is present. These require medical assessment rather than self-management, and several require emergency care rather than an appointment.

This list is not exhaustive. No list is. If something feels wrong, unexplained, or is changing quickly, get assessed regardless of whether it appears here.

How clinicians think about this

Musculoskeletal pain is common. Serious pathology presenting as musculoskeletal pain is uncommon. The job is not to be frightened of the rare thing, it is to have a system that reliably catches it.

Most clinicians work through what is called a pathological sieve: a fixed list of disease categories run through in order, so that nothing gets forgotten simply because it did not come to mind. The most widely used version is VITAMIN CDEF. It is worth you understanding it, because it tells you what a thorough clinician is quietly ruling out while they talk to you.

	Category	What raises suspicion
V	Vascular	Exertional pain eased by rest, pulsating abdominal or back pain, calf swelling and warmth, colour or temperature change in a limb, sudden severe headache or neck pain with neurological features. Includes heart attack, aortic aneurysm and dissection, deep vein thrombosis, pulmonary embolism and stroke. For the neck, screen with the 5 Ds, 3 Ns and 1 A: dizziness, diplopia (double vision), dysarthria (slurred speech), dysphagia (difficulty swallowing), drop attacks, nausea, numbness, nystagmus (flickering eye movements) and ataxia (loss of coordination). For stroke, BE-FAST: balance, eyes, face, arms, speech, time.

	Category	What raises suspicion
I	Infective and inflammatory	Fever, night sweats, rigors, recent infection or dental work, intravenous drug use, immunosuppression, recent spinal procedure. Also the inflammatory arthritides: morning stiffness beyond thirty to sixty minutes, better with movement and worse with rest, several joints, eye, skin or bowel involvement
T	Traumatic and toxic	Significant mechanism, inability to weight bear, deformity, or minor trauma in someone with osteoporosis or on long-term steroids. Also alcohol and drug effects
A	Autoimmune	Family history, multiple systems involved, symptoms that fluctuate in flares, associated fatigue, rashes, mouth ulcers or dry eyes
M	Metabolic	Diabetes and insulin resistance, gout, osteomalacia, electrolyte disturbance, obesity-related loading. Slow tissue repair and disproportionate pain sensitivity
I	Iatrogenic and idiopathic	Caused by treatment itself. Long-term steroids, statin-related muscle pain, post-surgical change, medication interactions. Idiopathic means no cause has been found, which is not the same as no cause existing
N	Neoplastic	Cancer, primary or secondary. Past history of any cancer, unexplained weight loss, new unexplained pain over the age of fifty, night pain unrelieved by any position, a new lump, progressive pain that does not vary with activity
C	Congenital	Present from birth. Hypermobility syndromes, structural anomalies, connective tissue disorders. Often explains why someone has had recurrent problems since adolescence
D	Degenerative	Osteoarthritis, disc degeneration, spondylosis, tendinopathy, sarcopenia. The most common category by far in musculoskeletal practice, and the one most often assumed without the others being excluded first
E	Endocrine and environmental	Thyroid disease, parathyroid disorders, menopause and hormonal change, vitamin D deficiency. Environmental exposures and occupational loading
F	Functional	Where structure is intact but function is not. Movement pattern problems, breathing pattern disorders, central sensitisation. Common, treatable, and a diagnosis of reasoning rather than exclusion

Notice where degenerative sits. It is the category most people are given, and it is third from last on the list. A good clinician arrives at it having considered the others, not instead of considering them.

Emergency: call 999 or go to A&E now

Cardiac. Chest pain, tightness or heaviness, particularly with breathlessness, sweating, nausea, or pain radiating to jaw, neck, or either arm. Shoulder or upper back pain brought on by exertion and eased by rest.

Cauda equina. Any new difficulty passing urine or sense of incomplete emptying. Loss of the sensation of needing to go, or of urine or stool passing. New incontinence. Numbness or altered sensation in the saddle area, including whether wiping feels normal. New loss of genital sensation or erectile dysfunction with back pain. Weakness or numbness in both legs. One of these is enough. Do not wait to see if it settles.

Stroke or vascular. Sudden severe headache or neck pain unlike anything you have had before, particularly with dizziness, double or blurred vision, slurred speech, difficulty swallowing, or facial numbness.

Stroke: BE-FAST. Balance, sudden loss of balance or coordination. Eyes, sudden blurred, double or lost vision. Face, drooping on one side. Arms, weakness or drift on one side. Speech, slurred or muddled. Time, call 999 immediately. BE-FAST is the expanded version of the FAST test used in the NHS Act FAST campaign, and adds the balance and vision signs that FAST misses.

Aneurysm. Sudden severe tearing back or abdominal pain, particularly with a pulsating sensation, feeling faint, or in anyone over sixty with vascular risk factors.

Clot. Calf swelling, warmth, redness or tenderness, especially after travel, surgery or immobility. With breathlessness or chest pain, treat as an emergency.

Cord compression. Rapidly progressive weakness, or numbness affecting both sides of the body.

Urgent. Same day or next day medical assessment

Fever alongside spinal or joint pain, or a hot swollen joint. Severe unrelenting pain at rest or at night that no position eases. Unexplained weight loss with pain. New neurological symptoms that are progressing. Inability to weight bear following a fall, particularly with osteoporosis or long-term steroid use. Any new pain in someone with a previous cancer diagnosis. New or worsening symptoms in anyone immunosuppressed or using intravenous drugs.

Cervical myelopathy. Hand clumsiness, difficulty with buttons, zips or keys, dropping things. Unsteadiness or a wider walking base. Numbness in both hands. These are subtle, they are commonly attributed to ageing, and prognosis worsens significantly with delay.

Book with your GP

Morning stiffness lasting more than thirty to sixty minutes, especially with pain that improves with movement and worsens with rest, or that wakes you in the second half of the night. Any new lump. Persistent change in bowel or bladder habit. Night sweats. Pain steadily worsening over weeks with no mechanical explanation. New eye redness or pain, mouth ulcers, psoriasis or bowel symptoms alongside joint pain. Widespread pain with profound fatigue. Any symptom that is new, unexplained and not settling.

If in any doubt at all, get checked. Being wrong about this costs you an appointment. Being wrong the other way costs considerably more.

The self-assessment checklist

This is close to the full set of questions I work through in a first consultation. Work through it before your next appointment, write the answers down, and hand them over. It is designed to surface precisely the information that normally gets missed.

The presenting complaint

- What happened, when, and how? Include the first mild version, not just when it became a problem
- How is it affecting your day to day life and function?
- Is it getting better, worse, or staying the same?
- Any neurological symptoms: numbness, tingling, weakness, loss of coordination
- Any associated symptoms at all, even if they seem unrelated
- Quality and nature of the pain: sharp, dull, burning, aching, throbbing
- Have you had this before, and what happened then?
- What makes it better, and what makes it worse?
- Previous history of pain and what interventions were tried
- Pain out of ten now, at worst, and at best
- Daily pattern across twenty-four hours
- Your occupation and what it physically demands
- What you expect from treatment, and what your concerns and beliefs are about what has happened

Medical history

- Smoking and alcohol, current and past
- Accidents and injuries, including ones you consider long resolved
- Illnesses, including childhood and infections
- Surgeries, including dental
- All previous investigations: blood tests, X-ray, CT, MRI, ultrasound, and their actual results
- All medications, current and recent, including short courses
- All supplements with doses
- Family history
- Diet and nutrition
- Exercise, current and historical
- Lifestyle, work pattern and stress load

Systemic enquiry

These are the questions most commonly skipped, and they are where non-mechanical drivers show up.

- **Cardiovascular:** chest pain, palpitations, breathlessness, ankle swelling, blood pressure, dizziness on standing
- **Respiratory:** cough, wheeze, breathlessness, breathing pattern, asthma history
- **ENT:** hearing, tinnitus, vertigo, sinus and nasal symptoms, sore throat, hoarseness, swallowing
- **Endocrine:** temperature tolerance, weight change, hair and skin changes, energy, thyroid history, menstrual cycle, menopause status
- **Gastrointestinal:** reflux, bloating, pain related to meals, food intolerances, appetite
- **Bowel and bladder:** frequency, urgency, consistency, blood, nocturia, any change from your normal
- **Urogenital:** pain, discharge, sexual function, pregnancy history

- **Psychosocial:** mood, anxiety, stress load, major life events, support, sleep quality
- **General:** headaches, vision, hearing, tinnitus, fevers, night sweats, unexplained weight change, bruising, energy compared with three years ago, general sense of wellbeing
- **Anything else:** do you think I have missed anything, or is there anything else you would like to share with me?

This is not an exhaustive list and no list is. Jaw pain, for example, is not on it. That last question is there because the thing that matters most is often the thing nobody thought to ask about.

Your four stress scores, out of ten

- Psychological and emotional load
- Inflammatory load
- Circadian and sleep disruption
- Blood sugar regulation

Before you leave the appointment

- Is there anything else at all you have not mentioned? Ask yourself this properly. It is remarkable how often the most important detail surfaces here
- Do you understand the diagnosis well enough to explain it back in your own words?
- Do you know what the plan is, what you are expected to do, and by when?

NEXT STEPS

Working with me

If you have read this far, something in it has probably matched your own experience.

The purpose of this guide was not to diagnose you. It was to show you what a thorough investigation actually looks at, so that you can tell what has been missed and ask for it specifically.

If you want that investigation done properly, the starting point is a free twenty-minute call. There is no obligation and no sales process. You tell me what has been happening, what you have already tried, and what has not worked. I will tell you honestly whether I think I can help, and if I do not think I am the right person, I will tell you that too.

Scan to book your free twenty-minute discovery call

Or go to **thestrengthrecoveryclinic.com**

How I work

I see people in clinic in London, at home across all London boroughs, and online worldwide. Consultations combine osteopathic assessment and treatment with a functional medicine approach to the systemic factors covered in Part Two, alongside rehabilitation, movement retraining and lifestyle guidance.

Online work is not a lesser version of this. In many cases it is more effective, because the time goes into the history, the investigation, movement retraining and the systemic drivers rather than into treatment on a couch. Needing someone's hands on you is not at the core of getting better.

Where private laboratory testing is genuinely likely to change what we do, I can arrange it. Where it is not, I will say so.

I work with a small number of people at a time. This is not a volume practice and it is not the right fit for everyone. If you are looking for a single session to sort everything out, or for someone to click your back and send you on your way, this will not suit you.

If you have been through the system, are tired of being managed rather than investigated, and are prepared to look at the whole picture rather than just the painful area, that is exactly the work I do.

Thank you for reading. Jean